Nursing & Health Survival Guide

Gerontological Care

Claire Welford

T0061944

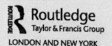
Routledge
Taylor & Francis Group

LONDON AND NEW YORK

First published 2013 by Pearson Education Limited

Published 2014 by Routledge
2 Park Square, Milton Park, Abingdon, Oxon OX14 4RN
711 Third Avenue, New York, NY 10017, USA

Routledge is an imprint of the Taylor & Francis Group, an informa business

ISBN 13: 978-0-273-77368-9 (hbk)

British Library Cataloguing-in-Publication Data
A catalogue record for this book is available from the British Library
Library of Congress Cataloging-in-Publication Data
Welford, Claire, author.
  Gerontological care / Claire Welford. – 1st edition.
    p. ; cm. – (Nursing and health survival guide)
  Includes bibliographical references.
  ISBN 978-0-273-77368-9 (pbk.)
  I. Title. II. Series: Nursing & health survival guides.
  [DNLM: 1. Geriatric Nursing–methods–Handbooks. WY 49]
  RC954
  618.97'0231–dc23

Typeset in 8/9.5pt Helvetica by 35

contents

As the world population ages and people live longer, nurses, regardless of which area they work in, will encounter older people. This book aims to provide nurses with the basic but fundamental knowledge that they will need to care for these older people.

Global statistics reveal a steady increase in the age of the world's population. In the USA it is estimated that by 2020 35 million people will be over 65 years of age and 7 million people will be over 85 years of age. Thus between 1990 and 2020 the population in the USA aged between 65 and 74 is projected to grow by 74%. In Australia 13% of the population were aged 65 and over in 2004. Those over 85 represented 1.5% of the Australian population and this is estimated to increase to 2–3% by 2021. The Swedish population of over-65s in 2000 was 23% and this is expected to increase to 31% by 2050. In the UK 20 million people were over 50 years of age in 2003 and this is projected to increase to 27.2 million by 2031. In Ireland the age of the population is also growing: in 2009, 13.14% of its population was over 65 (495,000 people) and this is estimated to increase to 22.4% by 2041.

Ageism

In 1973, Robert Butler and Myrna Lewis used the term ageism to describe 'a process of systematic stereotyping or discrimination against people because they are old, just as racism and sexism accomplish this with skin or gender'.

Wade (1999: 342) stated that, historically, the images portrayed of caring for older people have done little to create positive attitudes about caring for this client group. Furthermore, nurses themselves working in this speciality often have an 'inferiority complex' and feel 'isolated, undervalued and less glamorous' than their colleagues in other specialities. Wade (1999) concluded that staff need to be empowered, encouraged and educated to meet the care needs of older people and this will in turn create a shift in attitudes.

Randers and Mattiasson (2004) stated that research has shown that healthcare professionals' values, beliefs and attitudes towards older patients affect how they view and approach the patients in their care.

Katz (1960) defined an attitude as an individual predisposition to evaluate a symbol, object or aspect of the individual's world as positive or negative. Wesley (2005) stated that attitudes shape individuals' ability to understand, organise and clarify the world around them and influence the individual's behaviour and knowledge acquisition. More recently, Mandy, Lucas and Hodgson (2007) explained that attitudes may be considered to be a combination of positive and negative evaluations by which we interpret events, situations and relationships. Attitudes are based on our own experience of what others have told us, or what others have patterned for us.

Public awareness or representation of ageing issues may also impact upon society's level of understanding of ageing. Mandy, Lucas and Hodgson (2007) stated that the way older people are perceived publicly needs to be addressed.

Kogan (1961) developed an 'Attitude Scale' which is shown here. You might like to check your own attitudes on Kogan's Attitude Scale.

Kogan's Attitudes Towards Old People Scale

Directions: Circle the **letter** on the scale following each statement, according to the following key, that is closest to your opinion of old people. The range of scores is 34 to 204, with higher scores representing a more positive attitude. A=1 for positive statements (count from left to right) and A=6 for negative statements (count from right to left).

Key:

Strongly disagree	Slightly disagree	Disagree	Agree	Slightly agree	Strongly agree
A	B	C	D	E	F

1. It would probably be better if most old people lived in residential units with people their own age.

   A   B   C   D   E   F

2. There is something different about most people; it's hard to find out what makes them tick.

   A   B   C   D   E   F

3. People grow wiser with the coming of old age.

   A   B   C   D   E   F

4. Most old people get set in their ways and are unable to change.

    A   B   C   D   E   F

5. Most old people would prefer to quit work as soon as pensions or their children can support them.

    A   B   C   D   E   F

6. Most old people tend to let their homes become shabby and unattractive.

    A   B   C   D   E   F

7. Most old people are very relaxing to be with.

    A   B   C   D   E   F

8. Old people have too much power in business and politics.

    A   B   C   D   E   F

9. Most old people make one feel uneasy.

    A   B   C   D   E   F

10. It would probably be better if most people lived in residential units with younger people.

    A   B   C   D   E   F

11. Most old people are capable of new adjustments when the situation demands it.

    A   B   C   D   E   F

12. Most old people bore others by their insistence on talking about the 'good old days'.

    A   B   C   D   E   F

13. Most old people spend too much time prying into the affairs of others and giving unsought advice.

    A   B   C   D   E   F

14. Most old people can generally be counted on to maintain a clean, attractive home.

    A   B   C   D   E   F

▶

15. Old people should have power in business and politics.

    A   B   C   D   E   F

16. If old people expect to be liked, their first step is to try to get rid of their irritating faults.

    A   B   C   D   E   F

17. Most old people would prefer to continue working just as long as they possibly can rather than be dependent on anybody.

    A   B   C   D   E   F

18. In order to maintain a nice residential neighbourhood, it would be best if not too many old people lived in it.

    A   B   C   D   E   F

19. There are a few exceptions, but in general most old people are pretty much alike.

    A   B   C   D   E   F

20. Most old people should be more concerned with their personal appearance; they're too untidy.

    A   B   C   D   E   F

21. Most old people need no more love and reassurance than anyone else.

    A   B   C   D   E   F

22. Most old people are irritable, grouchy, and unpleasant.

    A   B   C   D   E   F

23. One of the most interesting and entertaining qualities of most old people is their accounts of their past experiences.

    A   B   C   D   E   F

24. It is foolish to claim that wisdom comes with age.

    A   B   C   D   E   F

25. Most old people are really no different from anybody else; they're as easy to understand as younger people.

   A   **B**   **C**   **D**   **E**   **F**

26. Most old people are cheerful, agreeable and good humoured.

   A   **B**   **C**   **D**   **E**   **F**

27. Most old people tend to keep to themselves and give advice only when asked.

   A   **B**   **C**   **D**   **E**   **F**

28. Most old people are constantly complaining about the behaviour of the younger generation.

   A   **B**   **C**   **D**   **E**   **F**

29. You can count on finding a nice residential neighbourhood when there is a sizeable number of old people living in it.

   A   **B**   **C**   **D**   **E**   **F**

30. When you think about it, old people have the same faults as anybody else.

   A   **B**   **C**   **D**   **E**   **F**

31. It is evident that most old people are very different from one another.

   A   **B**   **C**   **D**   **E**   **F**

32. Most old people make more excessive demands for love and reassurance than anyone else.

   A   **B**   **C**   **D**   **E**   **F**

33. Most old people seem quite clean and neat in their personal appearance.

   A   **B**   **C**   **D**   **E**   **F**

34. One seldom hears old people complaining about the behaviour of the younger generation.

   A   **B**   **C**   **D**   **E**   **F**

Adapted with permission from Kogan, N. (1961) Attitudes toward old people. The development of a scale and an examination of correlates, *Journal of Abnormal and Social Psychology*, 62(1), pp. 44–54.

Nursing assessment for the physiological changes associated with ageing

The first assessment performed by the nurse will no doubt take place immediately as he or she observes the dress, presentation and outer cleanliness of the older person.
It is important for the nurse to be aware of both normal and abnormal physiological changes as a result of ageing (Table 1).

Nursing assessment for elder abuse

In addition to assessing the older person's physiological health, the nurse must also assess for their safety. Assessing an older person's safety may be dependent on the relationship which the nurse may have with the older person. Trust is an integral ingredient in eliciting the required information. Both personal and home safety are major causes of concern for older people. Observing for signs of **elder abuse** is essential. There are eight types of abuse which the healthcare practitioner should be aware of:

- Physical
- Sexual
- Psychological
- Financial or material
- Neglect or acts of omission
- Discriminatory
- Social
- Emotional.

Table 1 Physiological changes associated with ageing

SKIN	MUSCULOSKELETAL	CIRCULATORY	SENSORY	RESPIRATORY	GASTROINTESTINAL
Epidermis thickens and dermis shrinks (dermal cells replaced more slowly). Less cell turnover. Decline in collagen and elastin levels.	Joint structures and ligaments increase in calcification and decrease in elasticity. Osteoarthritis is wear and tear and breakdown of the joints.	Heart decreases in weight due to increase of lipofuchsin in the myocardial fibres.	Decreased taste and saliva production.	Decrease in lung elasticity. Increase in chest wall stiffness. Decline in strength of respiratory muscles.	The epithelium that lines the digestive tract becomes thinner.
Hair loss from head and body but may increase in men in ears and nasal cavities.	Loss of bone mineral density: observe for osteoporosis (porous bones). Firstly, degeneration of the skeleton (osteopenia). Less exercise gives rise to bone loss.	Heart grows slightly larger and heart rate slows down. The arteries become filled with fatty deposits, 'atherosclerosis', which increases resistance to blood flow.	Progressive loss of higher sound frequency. Sounds are less clear and lower in volume.	Reduction in the surface area of the alveoli means that it takes more respiratory effort to complete the activities of living.	The stomach produces less hydrochloric acid, which reduces the absorption of calcium, iron, zinc and folic acid.

Table 1 *(cont'd)*

SKIN	MUSCULOSKELETAL	CIRCULATORY	SENSORY	RESPIRATORY	GASTROINTESTINAL
Decline in subcutaneous fat which can lead to hollowed cheeks and eye sockets.	Blood supply is less plentiful leading to muscle fatigue.	Usually normal red cells. White cell count tends to decrease. Clot reaction time may diminish in the platelets. Rise in ESR.	Memory disturbances.	Decrease in cough reflex leads to higher susceptibility of chest infections.	Peristalsis and bowel motility slow down, which can lead to constipation.
Blood vessels become more fragile.		Blood viscosity may increase without change in plasma.	Sensory receptors in the skin transmit sensations less rapidly. Also decrease in thyroid function leads to an unawareness of temperatures		Liver size and blood flow decrease, leading to a reduction in drug clearance ability.

SKIN	MUSCULOSKELETAL	CIRCULATORY	SENSORY	RESPIRATORY	GASTROINTESTINAL
Sweat output decreases. Skin becomes dry due to reduced activity of skin cells which produce natural oils. Incontinence may affect the skin.		Blood vessels lose their elasticity and subsequently blood pressure changes. Also more susceptible to postural hypotension as blood pressure falls much more on standing than when younger.	Visual acuity, colour differentiation, night vision and near vision all decline with age. Cataracts are formed when the lens of the eye gradually loses its natural transparency. Glaucoma occurs when fluid pressure within the eyeball is too high. Macular degeneration is caused by breakdown in the central part of the eye.		

Lachs and Pilemer (2004: 1264) defined elder abuse as:

> *'Intentional actions that cause harm or create serious risk of harm (whether or not harm is intended) to a vulnerable elder by a caregiver, or other person who stands in a trust relationship to the elder'.*

The signs of abuse are detailed in Table 2.

Nursing assessment of safety

Further to 'elder abuse', the older person's safety is also reduced by their increasing frailty and their decreasing sensory ability. Frequent vision and hearing tests are advised even if there are no complaints of deficits to either. The nurse should liaise with the multi-disciplinary team. Reduction of hazards at the primary point of care can clearly reduce accidents, thus preventing the need for secondary and tertiary care while simultaneously maintaining the person's independence for longer.

Safety assessments include assessment of:
- Perceived functional ability
- Fear in relation to falling
- Gait
- Mobility
- Muscle weakness
- Presence of osteoporosis
- Any cognitive impairment
- Incontinence
- Cardiovascular status.

The nurse may be the only person to whom the older person has to confide their worries, thus eliciting this information is

Table 2 The signs of elder abuse

PHYSICAL	SEXUAL	PSYCHOLOGICAL	FINANCIAL	NEGLECT
Bruises, lacerations, abrasions, scratches, burns, sprains, fractures, dislocations, marks left from a gag, hair loss, missing teeth and eye injuries.	Trauma to genitals, breasts, rectum, mouth. Injury to face and neck, chest, abdomen, thighs and buttocks. STDs or bite marks. Change in behaviour, social reluctance, nightmares, depression, sexually aggressive or inappropriate seductive behaviour, fear of being left alone with a particular person.	Demoralisation, depression, feelings of hopelessness or helplessness, tearfulness, agitation, resignation, confusion, unexplained paranoia.	Sudden inability to pay bills, sudden withdrawal of money from accounts, funds diverted for someone else's use, damage to property, disappearance of possessions, no funds for clothes, food or services, refusal to spend money, making dramatic financial decisions.	Dehydration, malnutrition, inappropriate clothing, poor hygiene, unkempt appearance, pressure sores, unattended medical needs, absence of required aids, e.g. glasses or dentures.

an integral part of the nursing assessment and contributes to providing high quality holistic care. Worries and fears may also have a profound effect on the older person's appetite.

Nursing assessment of nutritional status

Nutritional status may drop considerably as the person ages. Eating and drinking is an integral part of human life and an adequate intake of food and water is required to maintain physiological function, to allow for growth and maintenance of tissues and to provide energy to meet the demands of daily living.

The six main nutrient groups are as follows:

- **Proteins** are required for structure, movement, transport, immunity, acid–base regulation and osmotic pressure.
- **Carbohydrates** are required for energy, glucose energy for the brain and fibre production.
- **Lipids** are required for storing and providing energy, insulating beneath the skin and supporting and cushioning the organs.
- **Vitamins** are required for the body to grow and develop normally. The body needs 13 vitamins: vitamins A, C, D, E, K and the B vitamins (thiamine, riboflavin, niacin, pantothenic acid, biotin, vitamin B-6, vitamin B-12 and folate).
- **Minerals** are required for the body to stay healthy. The body uses minerals for many different jobs, including building bones, making hormones and regulating the heartbeat.

- **Water** is required for keeping the body temperature normal, lubricating and cushioning the joints, protecting the spinal cord and other sensitive tissues and getting rid of wastes through urination, perspiration, and bowel movements.

The Recommended Daily Allowances (RDA) for nutritional intake are shown in Table 3.

Table 3 Recommended Daily Allowances (RDA) for nutritional intake

	BOYS 9–13	BOYS 14–18	GIRLS 9–13	GIRLS 14–18
Calories	1,800–2,200	2,200–2,400	1,600–2,000	2,000
Protein (g)	34	52	34	46
Fat (g)	62–85	61–95	62–85	55–78
Saturated fat (g)	20–24	20	18–22	20
Cholesterol (mg)	<300	<300	<300	<300
Salt (g)	5	6	5	6
Sodium (mg)	1,500–1,900	1,500–2,300	1,500–2,200	2,300
Iron (mg)	8	11	8	15
Calcium (mg)	1,300	1,300	1,300	1,300
Fibre (g)	25–31	31–34	23–28	23
Vitamin A (mg)	500	600–700	500	600–700
Vitamin C (mg)	30	35–40	30	35–40
Folate (mg)	150–200	200	150–200	200
Calories	2,000–2,800	2,200–2,500	1,400–1,600	

Table 3 (cont'd)

	ADULTS 19–50	ADULTS 50 AND OVER	BOYS AND GIRLS 4–8
Protein (g)	55	53	19
Fat (g)	55–95	55–78	39–62
Saturated fat (g)	24–27	24–27	16–18
Cholesterol (mg)	<300	<300	<300
Salt (g)	6	6	3
Sodium (mg)	1,500–2,300	1,500–2,300	1,200–1,900
Iron (mg)	14.8	9	10
Calcium (mg)	1,300	1,300	800
Fibre (g)	31–34	31–34	19–23
Vitamin A (mg)	600–700	600–700	400
Vitamin C (mg)	35–40	35–40	30
Folate (mg)	200	200	100

Source: After the Food Standards Agency Nutrient and Food Based Guidelines for the UK, October 2007

There are several factors which may alter an older person's nutritional status, including socio-economic (reduced income due to retirement), disease processes associated with ageing, oral factors (reduced saliva production and/or weight loss causing dentures to become loose), reduced manual dexterity for preparing food, malabsorption, and diminished sensory ability (reduced levels of hunger and thirst, sight, sound and smell impairment).

In summary, a **nutritional assessment** of an older person should involve an assessment of the following:

- Normal eating habits
- Weight/body mass index (BMI) (Figures 1 and 2)
- Known medical conditions
- Dental condition
- Medications
- Activity levels
- Appetite
- Gastrointestinal factors
- Bladder/bowel habit
- Economic situation
- Physical/sensory/cognitive factors.

SI units	$BMI = \dfrac{\text{weight (kg)}}{\text{height}^2 \ (m^2)}$
Imperial units	$BMI = \dfrac{\text{weight (lb)} \times 703}{\text{height}^2 \ (in^2)}$
	$BMI = \dfrac{\text{weight (lb)} \times 4.88}{\text{height}^2 \ (ft^2)}$

Figure 1 Calculate your BMI

BMI RATING	STATUS
Below 20	Underweight
20–24.9	Normal Weight
25–29.9	Overweight (Grade 1 Obesity)
30–40	Moderately Obese (Grade 2 Obesity)
Over 40	Severely Obese (Grade 3 Obesity)

Figure 2 BMI scores

Weight loss, lethargy, light-headedness, disorientation and loss of appetite are often viewed as being symptoms of disease rather than malnutrition.

It is important for the nurse to be aware of community schemes available such as meals-on-wheels and daycare centres which can aid in maintaining the older person's nutritional status. Prevention of malnutrition can aid the prevention of secondary diseases and/or disease progression

It is recommended that a validated nutritional assessment tool is also used. Examples include the **MUST** score (Malnutrition Universal Scoring Tool) and the **MNA** (Mini Nutritional Assessment).

Assessment of the older person also includes gathering information about their support networks. As an older person moves into retirement they face the loss of social connection and relationships that they have had throughout their working lives. As time goes on, the older person may also experience the death of their spouse, relatives or friends. All of this contributes to a change in their ability to participate socially. Hospital wards and corridors are ideal places to exhibit examples of positive ageing, e.g. awareness posters, art exhibitions, creative writing exhibitions, etc., and health promotion literature. A possible checklist for the social assessment of an older person is as follows:

- Family/friends/visitors
- Telephone/TV/radio/communication skills
- Nearest neighbour/shop/church
- Transport
- Hobbies/interests
- Member of any groups/committees
- Health professional involvement.

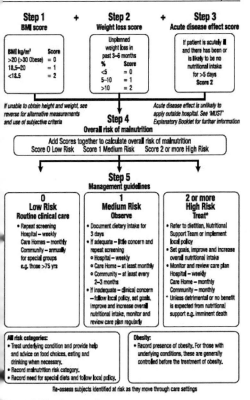

Step 1 + Step 2 + Step 3
BMI score **Weight loss score** **Acute disease effect score**

BMI kg/m²	Score
>20 (>30 Obese)	= 0
18.5–20	= 1
<18.5	= 2

Unplanned weight loss in past 3–6 months

%	Score
<5	= 0
5–10	= 1
>10	= 2

If patient is acutely ill and there has been or is likely to be no nutritional intake for >5 days

Score 2

If unable to obtain height and weight, see reverse for alternative measurements and use of subjective criteria

Acute disease effect is unlikely to apply outside hospital. See 'MUST' Explanatory Booklet for further information

Step 4
Overall risk of malnutrition

Add Scores together to calculate overall risk of malnutrition
Score 0 Low Risk   Score 1 Medium Risk   Score 2 or more High Risk

Step 5
Management guidelines

0 Low Risk
Routine clinical care

- Repeat screening
  Hospital – weekly
  Care Homes – monthly
  Community – annually
  for special groups
  e.g. those >75 yrs

1 Medium Risk
Observe

- Document dietary intake for 3 days
- If adequate – little concern and repeat screening
  ○ Hospital – weekly
  ○ Care Home – at least monthly
  ○ Community – at least every 2–3 months
- If inadequate – clinical concern – follow local policy, set goals, improve and increase overall nutritional intake, monitor and review care plan regularly

2 or more High Risk
Treat*

- Refer to dietitian, Nutritional Support Team or implement local policy
- Set goals, improve and increase overall nutritional intake
- Monitor and review care plan
  Hospital – weekly
  Care Home – monthly
  Community – monthly
- * Unless detrimental or no benefit is expected from nutritional support e.g. imminent death

All risk categories:
- Treat underlying condition and provide help and advice on food choices, eating and drinking when necessary.
- Record malnutrition risk category.
- Record need for special diets and follow local policy.

Obesity:
- Record presence of obesity. For those with underlying conditions, these are generally controlled before the treatment of obesity.

Re-assess subjects identified at risk as they move through care settings

Source: http://www.bapen.org.uk

Acute medical episodes in an older person's life can take many shapes and can stem from a failure to address some of the previously mentioned issues. There may also be signs of self-neglect. According to Pavlou and Lachs (2006), self-neglect in older adults is a complex phenomenon characterised by inattention to health and hygiene, typically stemming from an inability or unwillingness to access potentially remediating services.

Geriatric giants

Musso and Nuñez (2006) described three entities known as **geriatric giants**:

- Confusional syndrome
- Incontinence
- Gait disorders.

Some aspects of self-neglect clinically resemble these geriatric giants. These geriatric giants can appear as an acute event or as an exacerbation of an already existing state, often being the only clinical expression of various diseases such as pneumonia, urinary infection, cardiac infarction, etc. Possession of any combination of any two of these can be life-threatening for the older person, as one illness can impact or exacerbate the other.

■ CONFUSIONAL SYNDROME

Normal ageing processes may affect memory by changing the way in which the brain stores information and by making it harder to recall stored information. In addition, some age-related memory illnesses are categorised as confusional syndromes.

Dementia

Dementia refers to a group of cognitive illnesses characterised by a gradual and progressive impairment in memory, intellect, judgement, language and insight and a deterioration in social skills. Dementia is a condition in which there is a gradual loss of brain function; it is a decline in cognitive/intellectual functioning. The main symptoms are usually loss of memory, confusion, problems with speech and understanding, changes in personality and behaviour, and an increased reliance on others for the activities of daily living (Royal College of Psychiatrists).

The most common form of dementia in older people is vascular dementia, which tends to occur secondary to cardiac problems. Vascular dementia refers to a subtle, progressive decline in memory and cognitive functioning. It occurs when the blood supply carrying oxygen and nutrients to the brain is interrupted by a blocked or diseased vascular system. If blood supply is blocked for longer than a few seconds, brain cells can die, causing damage to the cortex of the brain (the area associated with learning, memory and language). Table 4 outlines the differences between vascular dementia and Alzheimer's disease.

Delirium

Delirium is an acute or sudden onset of mental confusion and rapid changes in brain function as a result of medical, social and/or environmental conditions. Signs of delirium include:

- Changes in cognitive function, e.g. worsened concentration, slow responses, confusion.
- Changes in perception, e.g. visual or auditory hallucinations.

Table 4 Key differences between Alzheimer's and dementi

SIGNS AND SYMPTOMS	VASCULAR DEMENTIA	ALZHEIMER'S DISEASE
Onset	Sudden	Gradual
Course	Stepwise progression, fluctuating	Gradual steady decline
Focal neurological changes	Present from outset	Develop in later stages
Memory loss	Milder, patchy, difficulty retrieving information	First sign, gradual loss of memory
Gait disorders	Early sign	Middle to late stages
Incontinence	Early sign	Middle to late stages
Personality	Remains intact longer	Gradual erosion
Emotional ability	More emotionally labile	Less emotionally labile
Depression	Common	Less common
Hallucinations and delusions	Common	Sometimes present, especially in later stages
Epileptic seizures	Seizures more likely at any stage	Seizures in later stages
Vascular risk and risk of sudden death	High risk of stroke, even unexpected death	Lower risk of sudden death

- Changes in physical function, e.g. reduced mobility, reduced movement, restlessness, agitation.
- Changes in appetite, and sleep disturbance.
- Changes in social behaviour, e.g. lack of cooperation with reasonable requests, withdrawal, or alterations in communication, mood and/or attitude.

Cognitive impairment

Cognitive impairment is a cognitive decline greater than expected for an individual's age and educational level. Cognition is the mental acquisition of knowledge through thought, experience and the senses.

Mental capacity is often determined by healthcare professionals through use of the Mini-Mental State Examination (MMSE), Figure 3. Folstein et al. (see p. 56) (1975) developed the Mini-Mental State Examination and stated that it is a brief neuropsychological test for evaluating cognitive status. MMSE scores are affected by age and education level, with lower scores being associated with increasing age and lower educational level. According to Dufouil et al. (2000), the norm for an 85-year-old man is 26 out of 30.

Care

When an older person suffers from a confusional syndrome, the nurse must aim to provide care which is person-centred: respecting the individuality of the person, their unique personality and their life experiences that influence their response to the disease.

The nurse must value the importance of the perspective of the person with dementia and the importance of their relationships and interactions with others.

Orientation to Time
"What is the date?"

Registration
"Listen carefully. I am going to say three words. You say
them back after I stop.
Ready? Here they are . . .
APPLE (pause), PENNY (pause), TABLE (pause). Now repeat
those words back to me." [Repeat up to 5 times, but score
only the first trial.]

Naming
"What is this?" [Point to a pencil or pen.]

Reading
"Please read this and do what it says." [Show examinee
the words on the stimulus form.]
CLOSE YOUR EYES

Figure 3 MMSE
Reproduced by special permission of the Publisher, Psychological Assessment
Resources, Inc., 16204 North Florida Avenue, Lutz, Florida 33549, from the
Mini-Mental State Examination, by Marshal F. Folstein, MD and Susan E. Folstein,
MD, Copyright 1975, 1998, 2001 by Mini Mental LLC, Inc. Published 2001 by
Psychological Assessment Resources, Inc. Further reproduction is prohibited
without permission of PAR, Inc. The MMSE can be purchased from PAR, Inc. by
calling (813) 968-3003.

People with dementia should have the opportunity to make informed decisions about their care and treatment in partnership with their health and social care professionals.

■ INCONTINENCE

It should not be assumed that all older people will become incontinent. However, there are normal physiological changes which can contribute to its occurrence:

- There is a slight decline in the bladder capacity so it cannot hold as much urine.
- The recognition of the need to pass urine does not occur until there is already more urine in the bladder than would be the case in a younger person, and as a result the urge is often felt too late.
- There is also a slight increase in the residual volume, which leads to an increase in the risk of a urinary tract infection (UTI).
- In women, the decrease in oestrogen can cause thinning of the urethral mucosa and a decline in muscle tone. Incontinence may be:
- Acute
- Transient
- Persistent.

Chronic incontinence may be of the following types:
- Stress
- Urge
- Overflow
- Functional.

Table 5 describes the symptoms of incontinence and suggests action plans.

Table 5 Common continence problems and action plans for reducing them

STRESS INCONTINENCE	ACTION PLAN	URGE INCONTINENCE	ACTION PLAN
Occurs when coughing, laughing or sneezing. Abdominal muscles tighten, thus raising the pressure on all the organs inside the abdomen including the bladder. Firm muscles around the sphincter will automatically exert a counter-pressure to prevent leakage. The pelvic floor muscles provide additional support.	Increase the tone of the pelvic floor muscles. Drug treatment.	Leakage of moderate to large volumes of urine immediately after a sudden and overwhelming urge to void. This happens because the detrusor muscle in the bladder contracts when it should not, possibly because the detrusor is hypersensitive or because normal neurological control has been lost, e.g. through stroke, Parkinson's, Alzheimer's or multiple sclerosis.	Reduce caffeine intake. Drink at least six half-pint glasses of non-caffeine fluids per day. Concentrate on increasing intervals between toileting. Antispasmodics and oestrogen preparations may help.

Table 5 (cont'd)

OVERFLOW INCONTINENCE	ACTION PLAN	FUNCTIONAL INCONTINENCE	ACTION PLAN
Accounts for less than 10% of incontinence in old age.	Remove any obstruction.	Cognitive dysfunction.	Requires comprehensive care planning.
Due to incomplete bladder emptying, resulting in retention.		Depression, leading to self-neglect.	
Leakage occurs when pressure from a chronically full bladder exceeds urethral pressure.		Immobility.	
		Difficulty in adjusting clothes.	
Overflow is often caused by an obstruction, e.g. constipation, prolapsed uterus or damage to the nervous system, or Benin Prostatic Hypertrophy (BPH) in men (dribbling, nocturia, urgency and frequency).		Lack of access to a toilet.	
		Excessive sedation.	

Urinary tract infections (UTI)

Urinalysis:

- Asymptomatic bacteriuria is common:
  - 15–30% in men
  - 25–50% in women.

How do we diagnose a UTI?

- Symptoms:
  - Dysuria, frequency, lower abdominal pain, urgency, haematuria
  - Absence of vaginal discharge or irritation.
- The probability of UTI in women is 90%.
- Urinalysis:
  - Pyuria.
- Mid-stream urine (MSU) sample.
- There is no evidence that an offensive odour correlates with UTI.
- There is no evidence that cloudy urine correlates with UTI.
- For a patient with dementia, is their behaviour different – are they restless or agitated?

For the asymptomatic patient:

- No treatment is required.
- A positive MSU probably represents asymptomatic bacteriuria
- Observe the patient.

For the symptomatic patient:

- Treat with appropriate antibiotics.

Long-term indwelling catheters (IDC):

- Long-term IDCs are always colonised.
- MSU/CSU may indicate which bacteria to treat if the patient becomes unwell.

- Ideally change the IDC just before CSU for the most accurate results.
- Treat if symptomatic: fever, loin pain.

Recurrent UTIs:
- Antibiotic prophylaxis is useful if more than three symptomatic UTIs per year or if patient is at risk of resistant organisms.

Constipation

Constipation is a common complaint among older adults. This is largely due to a decrease in bowel motility, reduced fluid intake, altered diet and reduced exercise. Constipation is defined as having a bowel movement fewer than three times per week. Constipation for the older person may be exacerbated by medications they are taking for other conditions. These include analgesia, anti-spasmodics, anti-Parkinson drugs and iron supplements.

Proactive rather than reactive management should occur:
- Encourage fluid intake.
- Take daily exercise.
- Increase dietary fibre.
- Encourage regular toileting.
- A diet with enough fibre (20 to 35 grams each day) helps the body form soft, bulky stools. High-fibre foods include beans, whole grains and bran cereals, fresh fruits, and vegetables such as asparagus, brussels sprouts, cabbage and carrots.

Different types of laxatives are available should the patient present with chronic constipation. However, it is important to note that the use of laxatives can also make the bowel sluggish, thus creating an increased need for further laxatives.

- **Bulk-forming laxatives** generally are considered the safest, but they can interfere with absorption of some medicines. These laxatives, also known as fibre supplements, are taken with water. They absorb water in the intestine and make the stool softer. These agents must be taken with water or they can cause obstruction. Many people also report no relief after taking bulking agents and suffer from a worsening in bloating and abdominal pain.
- **Stimulants** cause rhythmic muscle contractions in the intestines.
- **Osmotics** cause fluids to flow in a special way through the colon, resulting in bowel distention. This class of drugs is useful for people with idiopathic constipation. People with diabetes should be monitored for electrolyte imbalances.
- **Stool softeners** moisten the stool and prevent dehydration. These products are suggested for people who should avoid straining in order to pass a bowel movement. The prolonged use of this class of drugs may result in an electrolyte imbalance.
- **Lubricants** grease the stool, enabling it to move through the intestine more easily. Lubricants typically stimulate a bowel movement within 8 hours.
- **Saline laxatives** act like a sponge to draw water into the colon for easier passage of stools. Saline laxatives are used to treat acute constipation if there is no indication of bowel obstruction. Electrolyte imbalances have been reported and saline laxatives should therefore be used with caution in older people with renal deficiency.

■ GAIT DISORDERS

Older people should be assessed for the falls risk using an accredited tool, e.g. **FRASE** or **STRATIFY**.

RISK FACTOR	SCORE	ACTION	TICK/DATE
Male	1		
Female	2	Total score......	
AGE			
60–70	1	3–8 = LOW RISK	
71–80	2	9–12 = MEDIUM RISK	
81+	1	13+ = HIGH RISK	
GAIT			
Steady	0	See over for environmental/nurse action based	
Hesitant	1	on total score.	
Poor transfer	3		FRASE
Unsteady	3	If score > 1 on mobility/gait section refer to physiotherapy and OT. ⇒	
SENSORY DEFICIT			
Sight	2		
Hearing	1	If score > 1 on sensory deficit/medical section alert doctor to assess for reversible disease. ⇒	
Balance	2		
FALLS HISTORY			
None	0	If score =/> 1 on medications alert doctor/pharmacist	
At home	2	to consider rationalising medication. ⇒	
In ward	1		
Both	3	ALL ACTIONS TO BE RECORDED.	
MEDICATION			
Hypnotics	1		
Tranquillisers	1	ASSESS SCORE ON ADMISSION, ON TRANSFER TO	
Hypotensives	1	ANOTHER WARD, IN THE EVENT OF A SIGNIFICANT CLINICAL CHANGE AND ON DISCHARGE.	
MOBILITY			
Full	1		
Uses aid	2		
Restricted	3	RECORD SCORE ON DISCHARGE.	
Bed bound	1		
MEDICAL HISTORY			
Diabetes	1		
Dementia/Confusion	1		
Pits	1		

Adapted from Royal Bolton Hospital NHS Foundation Trust, http://www.bolton.nhs.uk/Library/services/med_manage/Osteoporosis_risk_treatment

Has the patient had a fall in the 4 weeks prior to admission or since admission to the residential home?
(Yes = 1, No = 0)

Do you think the patient is: (questions 2–5)

Agitated?
(Yes = 1, No = 0)

Visually impaired to the extent that their everyday function is affected?
(Yes = 1, No = 0)

In need of frequent toileting?
(Yes = 1, No = 0)

Gait pattern

Unable to walk/stand without major prompting and help? (Yes = 2)

Independently and safely mobile with or without a walking aid? (Yes = 0)

Mobile/independent with minimum assistance but unsteady? (Yes = 1)

Total Score

If a total score of 2 or more the patient is at risk of falling and will need appropriate care planned and delivered

STRATIFY

Adapted with permission from Folstein, M.F., Folstein, S.E. and McHugh, P.R. (1975) "'Mini-mental state'. A practical method for grading the cognitive state of patients for the clinician". *Journal of Psychiatric Research* 12(3), 189–98.

The risk of falling increases with age. About 30% of people aged over 65 years living in the community fall at least once a year; the fall rate is even higher in nursing homes. Many of these falls lead to fractures, the most serious type being hip fractures. There are multiple risk factors, including reduced vision, incontinence, reduced mobility, poor footwear, tripping hazards in the walking environment, changes in blood pressure leading to dizziness and imbalance, anaemia, living alone, and pain on exertion. The consequences of a fall are serious, for example fractures from osteoporotic bones, loss of confidence, further falls and increased falls risk, and may in fact mean that the older person can no longer stay living in their own home.

Falls as a result of medication are also common. The most common drug-related side-effects for older people are from anticholinergics (Mintzer and Burns 2000). Side-effects include insecure movements, falls without obvious reasons and blurred vision. Anticholinergics can affect memory and cause confusion and disorientation. Older people may be particularly susceptible to these side-effects because of their reduced metabolism and elimination and also age-related deficits in cholinergic neurotransmission. Antidepressants often result in sedation, leading to psychomotor retardation, and this is probably the main mechanism by which antidepressants cause falls. Adverse effects of antipsychotics include sedation, extrapyramidal problems and anticholinergic effects. All of the following could contribute to an increased risk of falls: sedation, leading to a slowing of psychomotor function; extrapyramidal gait disturbances; and anticholinergic-related visual blurring. Phenothiazines may also cause cataracts and the resultant poor vision could lead to falls. Anaemia is another cause of falls in older people (Penninx et al. 2005; Dharmarajan and Norkus 2004).

Management of falls

Management of falls needs to be multi-disciplinary and holistic. It includes comprehensive care planning for environmental, physical and physiological causes of falling (see Table 6).

Table 6 Falls prevention care planning: checklist for falls prevention

CLINICAL FACTORS (PHYSICAL AND PHYSIOLOGICAL)	ENVIRONMENTAL FACTORS
Abnormal blood results	Change in lighting
Infection	Ill-fitting footwear
Delirium	Unfamiliar/new surroundings
Dementia	Hazards
New medications	No call bell
Change in vision or hearing	
Parkinson's/TIA/CVA/MS	
Incontinence	

Other clinical concerns for older people

■ PRESSURE ULCERS

Pressure ulcers are defined as areas of localised damage to the skin and underlying tissue caused by pressure, shear, friction and/or a combination of these (European Pressure Ulcer Advisory Panel, EPUAP).

- Pressure ulcers are commonly referred to as bed sores, pressure damage, pressure injuries and decubitus ulcers.
- They require initial and on-going assessment of risk.
- They require initial and on-going pressure ulcer assessment

Risk assessment should be performed on admission using a validated tool such as those devised by Waterlow, Norton and Braden and shown here.

AREA SCORES IN TABLE, ADD TOTAL. MORE THAN 1 SCORE/CATEGORY CAN BE USED

BUILD/ WEIGHT FOR HEIGHT	◆	SKIN TYPE VISUAL RISK AREAS	◆	SEX AGE	◆	NUTRITION	
AVERAGE BMI (20–24.9)	0	HEALTHY	0	MALE	1	A – HAS PATIENT LOST WEIGHT RECENTLY	B – WEIGHT LOSS SCORE 0.5–5kg – 1
ABOVE AVERAGE BMI (25–29.9)	1	TISSUE PAPER DRY	1	FEMALE 14–49	1 1	YES – GO TO B	5–10kg – 2
OBESE BMI > 30	2	OEDEMATOUS CLAMMY, PYREXIA	1 1	50–64 65–74	2 3	NO – GO TO C UNSURE – GO TO C & SCORE 2	10–15kg – 3 >15kg – 4 UNSURE – 2
BELOW AVERAGE BMI > 20	3	DISCOLOURED STAGE 1	2	75–80 81+	4 5		
BMI = Wt/Ht (m²)		PRESSURE ULCER STAGE 2 – 4	3			C – PATIENT EATING POORLY/LACK OF APPETITE NO – SCORE 0 YES – SCORE 1	

CONTINENCE	◆	MOBILITY	◆	SPECIAL RISKS		
COMPLETE/ CATHETERISED	0	FULLY	0	TISSUE MALNUTRITION	◆	NEUROLOGICAL DEFICIT ◆
URINE INCONT.	1	RESTLESS/FIDGETY	1	TERMINAL CACHEXIA	8	DIABETES, MS, CVA 4–6
FAECAL INCONT.	2	APATHETIC	2	MULTIPLE ORGAN FAILURE	8	MOTOR SENSORY
URINARY + FAECAL INCONTINENCE	3	RESTRICTED	3	SINGLE ORGAN FAILURE (RESP, RENAL, CARDIAC.)	5	PARAPLEGIA (MAX OF 6)
		BEDBOUND E.G. TRACTION	4	PERIPHERAL VASCULAR DISEASE		
		CHAIRBOUND E.G. WHEELCHAIR	5	ANAEMIA (Hb < 8) SMOKING	2 1	MAJOR SURGERY OR TRAUMA
						ORTH-PAED/SPINAL 5 ON TABLE > 2 HR* 5 ON TABLE > 6 HR* 8

SCORE	
10 + AT RISK	
15 + HIGH RISK	
20 + VERY HIGH RISK	

MEDICATION
CYTOTOXICS, STEROIDS, ANTI-INFLAMMATORY MAX OF 4

Source: Judy Waterlow MBE SRN RCNT, http://www.judy-waterlow.co.uk, http://www.judy-waterlow.co.uk/the-waterlow-score-card.htm
Reproduced with permission.

Patient's Name _____		Evaluator's Name _____		Date of Assessment		
SENSORY PERCEPTION ability to respond meaningfully to pressure-related discomfort	**1. Completely Limited:** Unresponsive (does not moan, flinch, or grasp) to painful stimuli, due to diminished level of consciousness or sedation, OR limited ability to feel pain over most of body surface.	**2. Very Limited:** Responds only to painful stimuli. Cannot communicate discomfort except by moaning or restlessness, OR has a sensory impairment which limits the ability to feel pain or discomfort over 1/2 of body.	**3. Slightly Limited:** Responds to verbal commands, but cannot always communicate discomfort or need to be turned, OR has some sensory impairment which limits ability to feel pain or discomfort in 1 or 2 extremities.	**4. No Impairment:** Responds to verbal commands, has no sensory deficit which would limit ability to feel or voice pain or discomfort.		
MOISTURE degree to which skin is exposed to moisture	**1. Constantly Moist:** Skin is kept moist almost constantly by perspiration, urine, etc. Dampness is detected every time patient is moved or turned.	**2. Very Moist:** Skin is often, but not always, moist. Linen must be changed at least once a shift.	**3. Occasionally Moist:** Skin is occasionally moist, requiring an extra linen change approximately once a day.	**4. Rarely Moist:** Skin is usually dry, linen only requires changing at routine intervals.		
ACTIVITY degree of physical activity	**1. Bedfast:** Confined to bed.	**2. Chairfast:** Ability to walk severely limited or non-existent. Cannot bear weight and/or must be assisted into chair or wheelchair.	**3. Walks Occasionally:** Walks occasionally during day, but for very short distances, with or without assistance. Spends majority of each shift in bed or chair.	**4. Walks Frequently:** Walks outside the room at least twice a day and inside room at least once every 2 hours during waking hours.		
MOBILITY ability to change and control body position	**1. Completely Immobile:** Does not make even slight changes in body or extremity position without assistance.	**2. Very Limited:** Makes occasional slight changes in body or extremity position but unable to make frequent or significant changes	**3. Slightly Limited:** Makes frequent though slight changes in body or extremity position independently.	**4. No Limitations:** Makes major and frequent changes in position without assistance.		

usual food intake pattern	Never eats a complete meal. Rarely eats more than 1/3 of any food offered. Eats 2 servings or less of protein (meat or dairy products) per day. Takes fluids poorly. Does not take a liquid dietary supplement. OR is NPO and/or maintained on clear liquids or IV's for more than 5 days.	Rarely eats a complete meal and generally eats only about 1/2 of any food offered. Protein intake includes only 3 servings of meat or dairy products per day. Occasionally will take a dietary supplement. OR receives less than optimum amount of liquid diet or tube feeding.	Eats over half of most meals. Eats a total of 4 servings of protein (meat, dairy products) each day. Occasionally will refuse a meal, but will usually take a supplement if offered, OR is on a tube feeding or TPN regimen which probably meets most of nutritional needs.	Eats most of every meal. Never refuses a meal. Usually eats a total of 4 or more servings of meat and dairy products. Occasionally eats between meals. Does not require supplementation.	
FRICTION AND SHEAR	1. Problem: Requires moderate to maximum assistance in moving. Complete lifting without sliding against sheets is impossible. Frequently slides down in bed or chair, requiring frequent repositioning with maximum assistance. Spasticity, contractures or agitation lead to almost constant friction.	2. Potential Problem: Moves feebly or requires minimum assistance. During a move skin probably slides to some extent against sheets, chair, restraints, or other devices. Maintains relatively good position in chair or bed most of the time but occasionally slides down.	3. No Apparent Problem: Moves in bed and in chair independently and has sufficient muscle strength to lift up completely during move. Maintains good position in bed or chair at all times.		
				Total Score:	

Braden Pressure Ulcer Risk Assessment

Source: After © Barbara Braden and Nancy Bergstrom, 1988. Reprinted with permission. Permission should be sought to use this tool at www.bradenscale.com

The Norton tool is shown below.

Instructions: Complete the form by scoring each item from 1 to 4. Put 1 for low level of functioning and 4 for highest level of functioning.

Use: Use this tool in conjunction with **clinical assessment to determine if a patient is at risk for developing pressure ulcers.**

Pressure ulcer risk factors include:
- Pressure
- Shearing
- Friction
- Level of mobility
- Sensory impairment
- Continence
- Level of consciousness
- Acute, chronic and terminal illness
- Comorbidity
- Posture
- Cognition, psychological status
- Previous pressure damage
- Extremes of age
- Nutrition and hydration status
- Moisture to the skin.

Skin assessment should observe for:
- Persistent erythema
- Non-blanching hyperaemia
- Blisters
- Localised heat
- Localised oedema
- Localised induration

PHYSICAL CONDITION		MENTAL CONDITION		ACTIVITY		MOBILITY		INCONTINENCE		TOTAL SCORE
Good	4	Alert	4	Ambulant	4	Full	4	Not	4	4
Fair	3	Apathetic	3	Walk-help	3	Slightly limited	3	Occasional	3	3
Poor	2	Confused	2	Chair-bound	2	Very limited	2	Usually – urine	2	2
Very bad	1	Stupor	1	Stupor	1	Immobile	1	Doubly	1	1

Adapted from Norton, D., McLaren, R. and Exton-Smith, A. (1962) An Investigation of Geriatric Nursing Problems in the Hospital. London: Churchill Livingstone.

- Purplish/bluish localised areas
- Localised coolness if tissue death occurs.

Pressure ulcer grade should be recorded using the EPUAP classification system.

- **Grade 1**: Non-blanchable erythema of intact skin. Discolouration of the skin, warmth, oedema, induration or hardness can also be used as indicators, particularly on individuals with darker skin.
- **Grade 2**: Partial-thickness skin loss involving epidermis or dermis, or both. The ulcer is superficial and presents clinically as an abrasion or blister.
- **Grade 3**: Full-thickness skin loss involving damage to or necrosis of subcutaneous tissue that may extend down to but not through, underlying fascia.
- **Grade 4**: Extensive destruction, tissue necrosis, or damage to muscle, bone or supporting structures with or without full-thickness skin loss.

For patients with grade 1–2 pressure ulcers:

- As a minimum provision, patients should be placed on a high-specification foam mattress/cushion.
- Patients should be closely observed for skin changes.
- All pressure ulcers graded 2 and above should be documented as a local clinical incident.

For patients with grade 3–4 pressure ulcers:

- As a minimum provision, patients should be placed on a high-specification foam mattress with an alternating pressure overlay, or a sophisticated continuous low pressure system.
- The optimum wound-healing environment should be created by using modern dressings.

Treatment

Optimal management of a wound/pressure ulcer requires comprehensive and accurate assessment of wound history, aetiology recurrence and characteristics regarding location, staging, size, base, exudates and condition of surrounding skin.

Assessment for management should include:

- Cause
- Site/location
- Dimensions
- Stage or grade
- Exudate amount and type
- Local signs of infection
- Pain, including cause, level, location and management interventions
- Wound appearance
- Surrounding skin
- Undermining/tracking, sinus or fistula
- Odour
- Treatment should also include the following:
- Choose the dressing/topical agent or method of debridement or adjunct therapy based on:
  - ulcer assessment
  - general skin assessment
  - treatment objective
  - characteristic of dressing/technique
  - previous positive effect of dressing/techniques
  - manufacturer's indications/contra-indications for use
  - risk of adverse events
  - patient preference.
- Consider preventative measures, e.g. positioning, self-care, nutrition, pressure-relieving devices.

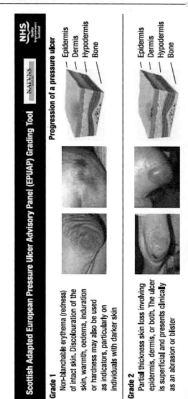

Scottish Adapted European Pressure Ulcer Advisory Panel (EPUAP) Grading Tool

Progression of a pressure ulcer

Epidermis
Dermis
Hypodermis
Bone

Epidermis
Dermis
Hypodermis
Bone

Grade 1

Non-blanchable erythema (redness) of intact skin. Discolouration of the skin, warmth, oedema, induration or hardness may also be used as indicators, particularly on individuals with darker skin

Grade 2

Partial thickness skin loss involving epidermis, dermis, or both. The ulcer is superficial and presents clinically as an abrasion or blister

Grade 3

Full thickness skin loss involving damage to or necrosis of subcutaneous tissue that may extend down to, but not through underlying fascia

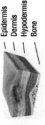

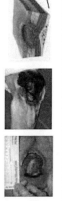

- Epidermis
- Dermis
- Hypodermis
- Bone

Grade 4

Extensive destruction, tissue necrosis, or damage to muscle, bone, or supporting structures with or without full thickness skin loss

- Epidermis
- Dermis
- Hypodermis
- Bone

www.tissueviabilityonline.com/pu

Source: NHS Quality Improvement Scotland, 2009

- Create an optimum wound-healing environment using modern dressings.
- Consider oral antimicrobial therapy in the presence of systemic and/or local clinical signs of infection.
- Consider referral to a surgeon.
- Consider mobilising, positioning and repositioning interventions for *all* patients.
- All patients with pressure ulcers should actively mobilise, change position or be repositioned.
- Minimise pressure on bony prominences and avoid positioning on pressure ulcers.
- Consider restricting sitting time.
- Seek specialist advice on aids, equipment and positions.
- Record using a repositioning chart or schedule.
- Provide nutritional support to patients with an identified deficiency.

Medications and older people

By their nature as substances with biological activity on the body, all medicines are associated with a risk of harming patients, ranging from minor risks to severe risks and from rare to common in their frequency of occurrence. The level of risk is dependent upon the drug properties, the administration route, concomitant medication, and patient factors such as drug levels in the body, age and gender. Prescription errors, over-prescribing and incorrect diagnosis also pose risks.

- **Pharmacodynamics** is the process by which the drug interacts with the body to bring about its effects ('What the drug does to the body').

- **Pharmacokinetics** is the process by which the body deals with the drug ('What the body does to the drug').

Pathological state

In older adults, renal function is frequently impaired. Impairments in renal function could have a dramatic effect on the pharmacokinetics of drugs that normally would be eliminated via the kidney. Consequently, such patients will tend to accumulate such drugs, and reductions in drug dose will often need to be considered. Some patients may have impaired liver function, which will result in decreased metabolic activity. In severe cases, this could result in dramatic changes in the plasma concentration of drugs that are ordinarily extensively metabolised.

Polypharmacy

Many older people are subject to polypharmacy. Polypharmacy has many definitions in the literature. Some define it as the use of two or more drugs for 240 days or more, others as the use of four or more medications, and still others as the use of five or more medications. This lack of consensus on a definition led Fulton and Allen (2005) to suggest a new definition:

Polypharmacy: 'the use of medications that are not clinically indicated'. Bilowski *et al.* (2001) suggested several ways in which polypharmacy can be reduced. These include adopting the '**brown bag**' approach whereby clients bring their prescription and non-prescription medications to their primary care provider who then reviews what they are taking. However, many adopt the '**Beers criteria**' which help clinicians to identify adverse reactions for medications that should be avoided or used cautiously in the older population. Others advocate the use of the **SAIL** and **TIDE** criteria:

- S: Keep the drug regimen *Simple* to once or twice daily dosing. Try to treat multiple symptoms and syndromes with a single drug that may have multiple beneficial effects, rather than treating each symptom or syndrome with individual drugs.
- A: Understand the potential *Adverse* effects.
- I: Each drug should have a clear *Indication* and a well-defined therapeutic goal.
- L: *List* the name and dosage of each drug on the client's chart.

- T: Allow *Time* for sufficient consultation.
- I: Apply *Individual* variability.
- D: *Drug*–drug interactions.
- E: *Educate* clients about their drugs.

There is also the Prescribing Optimisation Method (POM) which uses six questions to assist the healthcare provider in reducing polypharmacy:

- Is under-treatment present and is addition of medication indicated?
- Does the patient adhere to his or her medication schedule?
- Which drug(s) can be withdrawn or are inappropriate?
- Which adverse effects are present?
- Which clinically relevant interactions are to be expected?
- Should the dose, dose frequency and/or form of drug be adjusted?

Think point

Mary Goodridge is an older woman on many different medicines to manage her complex needs. One of her medicines is Ibuprofen for her knee pain. She is also on Warfarin for her atrial fibrillation. Using the BNF, identify any possible interactions between these drugs and consider a suitable alternative.

Look at the medicine charts/prescriptions of one of your patients. Are they receiving any unnecessary medications or doses?

CEREBROVASCULAR ACCIDENT (CVA) STROKE

Every year, an estimated 150,000 people in the UK have a stroke (Stroke Association 2012). A reduction of, or merely a disruption in, blood circulatory flow to the brain is the major contributory factor in a stroke.

The Department of Health (2009) recommends the acronym FAST for how to spot a stroke:

- Facial weakness: Can the person smile? Has their mouth or eye drooped?
- Arm weakness: Can the person raise both arms?
- Speech problems: Can the person speak clearly and understand what you say?
- Time to call 999.

The Bamford Oxford stroke criteria (Bamford *et al.* 1991) are used to classify strokes: see Table 7.

Initial management

The Royal College of Physicians (2008) states that everyone with an acute stroke who has not had primary intracerebral haemorrhage should be given 300 mg of aspirin as soon as possible and within 24 hours of the stroke.

A stroke can cut off or reduce oxygen levels to parts of the brain. The brain tissue that is suffering from reduced levels of

Table 7 The Bamford Oxford stroke criteria

	LACUNAR	PARTIAL ANTERIOR CIRCULATION	TOTAL ANTERIOR CIRCULATION	POSTERIOR CIRCULATION
Clinical signs and symptoms	Evidence of sensory or motor deficit only	Two or more of the following: Sensory deficit Motor deficit Higher cortical Dysfunction Hemianopia	All of the following: Sensory deficit Motor deficit Cortical Hemianopia	Any of the following: Isolated Hemianopia Brain stem signs Cerebellar ataxia

oxygen because of stroke may die. Improving oxygenation of tissues by monitoring oxygen saturation levels and giving oxygen provides high levels of oxygen to cells that have been damaged but not killed by the stroke. This reduces damage and improves the person's potential to recover. The RCP (2008) guidance recommends that oxygen should be given if oxygen saturation drops below 95%.

Ischaemic stroke may produce an acute rise in blood pressure, which can cause further stroke. The RCP guidance recommends that blood pressure is monitored and only treated in certain circumstances (RCP 2008).

The person may have a cardiac arrhythmia and may require cardiac monitoring and treatment. Cardiac arrthymias increase the risk of clots or emboli developing.

Stroke can affect temperature regulation and cause high temperatures. High temperature increases oxygen demands on all tissues including the brain. Paracetomol should be given to control high temperatures.

Stroke can affect blood sugar control. Specialist units should monitor blood sugar carefully and aim to maintain a blood glucose of between 4 and 11 mmol/litre.

Stroke can impair mobility. People who have a stroke should be sat up as soon as possible, sat out of bed and encouraged and assisted to move around as soon as possible (RCP 2008).

The RCP guidance (2008) recommends that people with acute stroke are screened for swallowing problems.

Approaches to gerontological care

Approaches to gerontological care are advancing and include care planning developments and care approaches.

■ CARE PLANNING

Comprehensive care for the older person requires the systematic and continuous collection of data. Subsequent to using validated assessment tools the nurse and the older person should compile the care plan.

There are many nursing models available which underpin care planning documentation. According to Pearson (1996), at a basic level there are three key components to a nursing model:

- A set of beliefs and values
- A statement of the goal the nurse is trying to achieve
- The knowledge and skills the nurse needs to practise.

Fawcett (1995) suggests that the central concepts are:

- Person: the recipient of nursing actions
- Environment: the recipient's specific surroundings
- Health: the wellness or illness state of the recipient
- Nursing: actions taken by nurses on behalf of or in conjunction with a recipient.
- The most commonly used nursing models are summarised in Table 8.

For successful care planning, the nurse (assessor) must take cognisance of the attributes the person brings with them in their current presentation (problem) and how this affects the future choices, in terms of both their ability to make them and the range of choices available. Hence the life history of the older person is particularly important for those in residential care. The older person's past life may shape their present life wishes. Tutton (2005) and Cook (2010) stated that understanding patients' personal histories and biographies creates opportunities for knowing what is

Table 8 Example of nursing models

NURSING MODEL	SUMMARY OF THE MODEL
Roper, Logan and Tierney Model	Describes the person as being capable of performing 12 activities of living along an independence–dependence continuum throughout the lifespan.
Orem's Model	Nurses would assess patients for their individual self-care deficits and plan an appropriate set of interventions to help them to overcome and restore their self-care deficits as much as possible.
Neuman's System Model	Emphasises the need to assess the patient for the stressors affecting them and provide appropriate interventions to offset the effects of these stressors.

important to them. It also provides an insight into how they are experiencing their present situations. Tutton (2005) reported that knowing the (authentic) person and how they would like to live their daily life provides the basis for participation in daily care.

■ PERSON-CENTRED CARE (PCC) IN NURSING HOMES

The theory of person-centred care evolved from a desire to create an approach to nursing home care that is non-paternalistic and non-task orientated. There has been an extensive amount of debate and discussion in the literature encouraging organisations to adopt a person-centred approach to care in nursing homes for older people (Manley and McCormack 2003; McCormack 2001, 2004).

Patient- or person-centred care (PCC) may be explained as care that is respectful of and responsive to individual patients' preferences, needs and values whilst ensuring that patient values guide all clinical decisions (Institute of Medicine 2001). Manley and McCormack (2003) explained that PCC is a term used to describe the therapeutic relationships between care providers and service users, and between care providers themselves.

The majority of papers published about person-centred care have focused on providing frameworks for clinical practice (McCormack 2004; McCormack and McCance 2006; Manley and McCormack 2003; Nolan *et al*. 2004; Ford and McCormack 2000; Titchen 2000). Many of these frameworks share similar recommendations for effective staff/resident communication, staff expertise in working with older people, a sense of humanity in the care environment, and the establishment and maintenance of successful staff/resident relationships.

The '**positive-person framework**' was developed by Kitwood (1990) and has its roots in social psychology. Kitwood (1990) stated that the approach to communication influences the type of caregiving and the culture of care.

Titchen (2000) then devised the '**skilled companionship**' theory, which stated that the nurse must possess a high level of expertise in knowing the older person in order to deliver PCC.

The **Burford Nursing Development Unit** in Oxfordshire developed a humanistic framework that facilitated nurses and residents to consider the lived experience.

Nolan *et al.* (2004) devised the 'senses framework', which focused on residents' need for security, belonging, continuity, purpose, achievement and significance. They suggested that the senses framework for PCC is actually dependent upon relationships.

McCormack (2001) aimed to further develop the PCC theory and stated that there are four concepts underpinning person-centred nursing:

- Being in relation
- Being in a social world
- Being in place
- Being with self.

Being in relation is about the relationship between the nurse and the patient. Being in a social world relates to knowing the person's social interests and devising life-plans for them. Being in place relates to the patient feeling a sense of place in the home, and being with self relates to private time being facilitated for the patient.

What all of these frameworks have in common is the recognition of the patient as central to the care relationship and that the patient has a personality shaped by their life experiences. However, Dewing (2004) argued that these frameworks need further development in order to make them meaningful for older people and for the nurses working with them.

In order to advance the use of these frameworks in practice, various prerequisites to PCC have more recently been presented in the literature. McCormack (2001) stated that getting close to the patient and building a relationship with them is the vital step required for achievement of PCC.

McCormack and McCance (2006) added that a PCC approach to care delivery requires prerequisites such as professionally competent staff, developed interpersonal skills, commitment to the job, clarification of values and beliefs, and knowing the self. The care environment needs an appropriate skill mix, a shared decision-making system, effective staff relationships, potential for innovation and risk taking, and supportive organisational systems.

Welford *et al.* (2010) identified the attributes of autonomy for older people in residential care and stated that resident autonomy must be present before person-centred care can be achieved. These attributes are:

- The capacity of residents is encouraged and maintained.
- Residents are involved in decision-making.
- Residents delegate care needs based on the right to self-determination and the rights of older people.
- Negotiated care plans are encouraged through open and respectful communication.
- The residential unit has a culture and atmosphere of flexibility within an ethos of maintaining residents' dignity.
- Family or significant others are included for residents who are cognitively impaired.

These theories and frameworks can be implemented into the older person's care plans in the ways shown below.

Care planning tips

- The process of care planning should be matched by what is documented in the care plans.
- **ASPIRE** is the new nursing process cycle: Assessment, Planning, Implementation, Re-check and Evaluation (Barrett *et al*, 2009).

- Link medical diagnosis with nursing diagnosis, e.g. due to John's Parkinson's he needs help with washing and dressing.
- Link assessment score into care plans, e.g. John's MUST score into his eating and drinking care plan.
- Describe how the resident/client/patient would like to spend their day.
- Start with a positive statement about the resident/client/patient strength, e.g. if you give John a basin of water he will wash his own hands and face.
- Identify actual and/or potential care issues.

You should aim for a person-centred care plan PRODUCT:

- Person-centred: Is the care plan goal tailored to the needs of the resident/client/patient?
- Recordable: Can you document the progress?
- Observable and measurable: Can you evaluate the progress?
- Directive: Who, what and how?
- Understandable: Is it written in a simple way?
- Credible: Can the goals be realistically achieved?
- Time related: When is the goal meant to be achieved?

End of life

Originally palliative care was developed as a method for caring for terminally ill cancer patients. The role of palliative care is increasing, being expanded to include other patients (older adults) facing the reality of their own imminent death.

Many older people have an advanced, progressive, life-limiting illness, their condition deteriorating over an extended period of time with a long lead time to death.

The *principles of palliative care* are as follows:

- A focus on quality of life
- Maintaining good symptom control
- A holistic approach which takes into account the person's life experience and current situation
- Care that encompasses the patient and those who matter to them, including support in bereavement
- Open and sensitive communication with residents, carers, families and professional colleagues.

Adopting a palliative approach to care throughout the older person's illness trajectory enables staff to move away from viewing palliative care as restricted to care of the dying person only.

The older person should receive comprehensive, compassionate end-of-life care that is person-centred and responds to their unique needs and respect for their wishes.

When older people are at the end of their lives, nurses can make a difference to them and their families by creating and facilitating a therapeutic milieu that addresses their physical, psychological, social, cultural and spiritual needs. This includes collaboration with other healthcare professionals in providing evidence-based best practice and establishing mechanisms for consultation regarding practice and referral. Older people may feel disempowered in their decision-making at this time. In order to protect their rights, it is important to be guided by, and to work within, a legal framework.

The nurse must maintain dignity, comfort and privacy for the older person throughout the end of life/dying process.

References

Bamford, J., Sandercock, P., Dennis, M., Burn, J. and Warlow, C. (1991) Classification and natural history of clinically identifiable subtypes of cerebral infarction. *The Lancet* 22, 337(8756), 1521–6.

Barrett D., Wilson B., Woolands, A. (2009) Care planning: A guide for nurses. Harlow: Pearson Education.

Bilowski, R.M., Rispin, C.M. and Lorraine, V.L. (2001) Physician patient congruence regarding medication regimens. *Journal of American Geriatrics Society* 49, 1353–7.

Butler, R., Sunderland, T. and Lewis, M. (1973) Aging and Mental Health: Positive Psychosocial and Biomedical Approaches. USA: Penguin Group.

Cook, G. (2010) Ensuring older residents retain their unique identity. *Nursing & Residential Care* 12(6), 290–3.

Department of Health (2009) available at www.dh.gov.uk.

Dewing, J. (2004) Concerns relating to the application of frameworks to promote person-centredness in nursing with older people. *Journal of Clinical Nursing* 13(1), 39–44.

Dharmarajan, T.S. and Norkus, E.P. (2004) Mild anemia and the risk of falls in older adults from nursing homes and the community. *Journal of the American Medical Directors Association*, November, 5(6), 395–400.

Dufouil, C., Clayton, D., Brayne, C., Chi, L.Y., Dening, T.R., Paykel, E.S., O'Connor, D.W., Ahmed, A., McGee, M.A. and Huppert, F.D. (2000) Population norms for the MMSE in the very old. Estimates based on longitudinal data. *Neurology*, December, 55(1), 1609–13.

Fawcett, J. (1995) *Analysis and Evaluation of Conceptual Models of Nursing*. Philadelphia, PA: FA Davis Co.

Folstein, M.F., Folstein, S.E. and McHugh, P.R. (1975) "'Mini-mental state'. A practical method for grading the cognitive state of patients for the clinician". *Journal of Psychiatric Research* 12(3), 189–98.

Ford, P. and McCormack, B. (2000) Contemporary approaches to nursing assessment with older people: the RCN Nursing Older People Assessment Tool. London: *Royal College of Physicians Newsletter*.

Fulton, M.M. and Allen, E.R. (2005) Polypharmacy in the elderly: a literature review. *Journal of the American Academy of Nurse Practitioners* 17, 123–32.

Institute of Medicine (2001) Crossing the quality chasm: A new health system for the 21st Century. Available at http://www.iom.edu/.

Katz, D. (1960) The functional approach to the study of attitudes. *Public Opinion Quarterly* 24, 163–204.

Kitwood, T. (1990) The dialectics of dementia: with particula reference to Alzheimer's disease. *Ageing and Society* 10, 177–96.

Kogan, N. (1961) Attitudes toward old people. The development of a scale and an examination of correlates. *Journal of Abnormal and Social Psychology* 62(1), 44–54.

Lachs, M.S. and Pilemer, K. (2004) Elder abuse. *The Lancet*, October, 364, 1263–72.

Mandy, A., Lucas, K. and Hodgson, L. (2007) Clinical educators' reactions to ageing. *International Journal of Allied Health Sciences and Practice* 5(4), 1–14.

Manley, K. and McCormack, B. (2003) Practice development: purpose, methodology, facilitation and evaluation. *Nursing in Critical Care* 8(1), 22–9.

McCormack, B. (2001) *Negotiating Partnerships with Older People: A Person-Centred Approach.* Aldershot: Ashgate.

McCormack, B. (2004) Person-centredness in gerontological nursing: an overview of the literature. *International Journal of Older People Nursing* 13(3a), 31–8.

McCormack, B. and McCance, T. (2006) Development of a framework for person-centred nursing. *Journal of Advanced Nursing* 56(5), 472–9.

Mintzer, J. and Burns, A. (2000) Anticholinergic side-effects of drugs in elderly people. *Journal of the Royal Society of Medicine,* September, 93, 457–62.

Musso, C.J. and Nuñez, J.F.M. (2006) Feed-back between geriatric syndromes: general system theory in geriatrics. *International Urology and Nephrology* 38(3–4), 785–6.

Nolan, M.R., Davies, S., Brown, J., Keady, J. and Nolan, J. (2004) Beyond 'person-centred' care: a new vision for gerontological nursing. *International Journal of Older People Nursing* 13(3a), 45–53.

Pavlou, M.P. and Lachs, M.S. (2006) Could self-neglect in older adults be a geriatric syndrome? *Journal of the American Geriatrics Society,* May, 54(5), 831–42.

Pearson, A. (1996) *Nursing Models for Practice.* Oxford: Butterworth-Heinemann.

Penninx, B., Pluijm, S., Lips, P., Woodman, R., Miedema, K., Guralnik, J. and Deeg, D. (2005) Late-life anemia is associated with increased risk of recurrent falls. *Journal of the American Geriatrics Society*, December, 53(12), 2106–11.

Randers, I. and Mattiasson, A.C. (2004) Autonomy and integrity: upholding older patients' dignity. *Journal of Advanced Nursing* 45(1), 63–71.

Royal College of Physicians (2008) available at www.rcpi.ie.

Stroke Association (2012) available at www.stroke.org.uk.

Titchen, A. (2000) *Professional craft knowledge in patient-centred nursing and the facilitation of its development*. D.Phil thesis, Linacre College, Oxford. Tackley, Oxfordshire: Ashdale Press.

Tutton, E.M.M. (2005) Patient participation on a ward for frail older people. *Journal of Advanced Nursing* 50(2), 143–52

Wade, S. (1999) Promoting quality of care for older people: developing positive attitudes to working with older people *Journal of Nursing Management* 7, 339–47.

Welford, C., Murphy, K., Casey, D. and Wallace, M. (2010) A concept analysis of autonomy for older people in residential care. *Journal of Clinical Nursing* 19, 1226–35.

Wesley, S.C. (2005) Enticing students to careers in gerontology: Faculty and student perspectives. *Gerontology & Geriatrics Education* 25(3), 13–29.